TRAIN. NOURISH. RECOVER.

16-WEEK TRAINING PLAN

RUNNING JOURNAL

MILES & MACROS

IMAGINEWE Publishers™

ImagineWe Publishers
A Global Publisher

IMAGINEWE
Publishers™

Published by ImagineWe, LLC
ImagineWe Publishers
247 Market Street, Suite 201
Lockport, NY 14094
United States
www.imaginewepublishers.com

ISBN: 978-1-946512-99-4 (Paperback)
ISBN: 979-8-9917997-0-6 (Hardback)

First Edition

To every runner who shows up for themselves.

Contents

HOW TO USE THIS JOURNAL

- Start from the back of the journal on week 16 on page 108. Write in the date of your race. Then begin to date your journal backwards 16 weeks. The date at the beginning of your journal, on page 22, is when to start your 16-week training for your goal race.
- A 16-week training plan is most commonly used for marathons and half marathons.
- You run six days a week:
    - Four runs a week are "base runs." These are conversational, easy pace runs.
    - One run a week is a "speed session." This is considered one day of quality.
    - One day is a rest day.
    - One run a week is a long run, normally done on a Saturday. The long run is a long, slow distance. You up your long runs 10% every two weeks.
- The habits pages are where you can write down your goals, intentions, or affirmations for the day or the future. This helps with focus and motivation.
- This journal is broken down into four training phases. Each training phase has different elements that make up the cycle.
    - In Phase 1 you lay down your foundational work (building your base).
    - In Phase 2 you practice running at a faster pace.
    - In Phase 3 you elevate your training for your specific race - think terrain and elevation.
    - And lastly, in Phase 4 you taper.
- **Self Care Tracker:** Did you take care of yourself throughout this phase? Self care is the most important care.

- **Training Notes:** How is training feeling? Do you have any issues, pains, questions, or achievements you want to document?
- **Mental Health Reflections:** Reflect on the entire phase you just completed, add any insights you gained or lessons learned.
- **Samples:** At the end of this journal, you will find a sample workout week and speed session.

About Miles & Macros:

This journal can be used with Miles & Macros coaching plans. Check out our website by scanning the QR code located at the end of the journal.

MEET YOUR TRAINER.

Hi, I am Lauren Burdick and I am a certified sports nutrition consultant, certified running coach, and co-owner of Miles & Macros, LLC (personal coaching for running, cycling, sports nutrition, and race directorsof three trail races located in Upstate New York).

I have had the pleasure of training runners who are just beginning their running journey to those runners completing the marathon distance. I believe my approach to coaching provides an understanding of consistent, daily training, enduring long periods of time out on race courses, and a woman's approach to running routines.

I have been running for over 12 years and enjoy distances ranging from 5k to ultra-marathons and running on road, track, or trail. Running has given me a sense of community, purpose, drive, and happiness. I began coaching because empowering and inspiring others to achieve their goals gives me a rush similar to the finish line of my race! I want to see others find a sense of community, health, and nutrition in a safe and effective way.

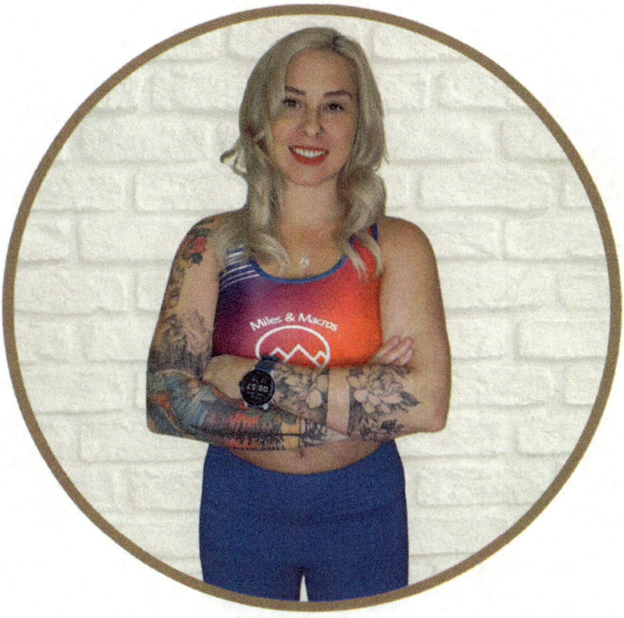

GOALS TRACKER

ENTER MONTHS & THE GOALS ACCOMPLISHED

YEAR: ______

GOALS TRACKER

RACE YEAR: _________

My Top Three Goals	
1	
2	
3	

Action Plan

PHASE 4

PHASE 3

PHASE 2

PHASE 1

Rewards	1	2	3	4

TRAIN. NOURISH. RECOVER.

HABIT TRACKER

Did you complete everything each week?

Color in the square under each week when you complete the following:

WEEKS:

Followed your training plan (6 runs a week)

Slept 8 hours each night of the week

Completed your daily mobility each week

Tuned in on your mental health each week

Drank 8 glasses of water per day each week

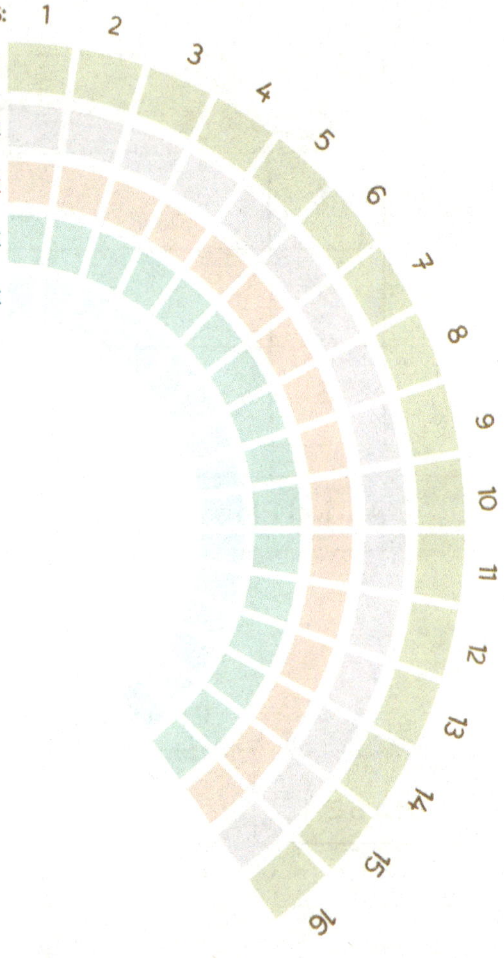

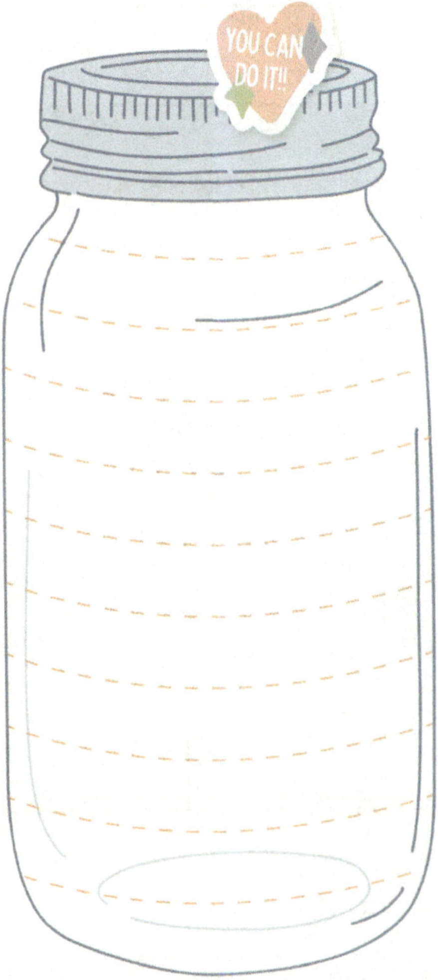

On each line in the mason jar write something you are proud of. Fill this jar with self-love throughout your 16-weeks!

PHASES EXPLAINED

	1	2	3	4	5
PHASE 1 - BASIC	○	○	○	○	○
PHASE 2 - SPEED DEVELOPMENT	○	○	○	○	
PHASE 3 - SPECIFIC	○	○	○	○	
PHASE 4 - TAPER	○	○	○		

This 16 week plan has 4 phases:

- Phase 1 is where you establish general conditioning. Think of this as building your foundation/preparing your base and preparing you for the work you will do ahead. It is important to go off of effort in this phase.
- Phase 2 is where you get better at running at higher speeds surrounding your goal race pace. This is a time to practice correlating effort to race pace.
- Phase 3 is the specific phase where you train for your race specifics (i.e. trail, hills, flat, road, elevation). This is where you want to work very close to race pace.
- Phase 4 is where you let your body absorb all the training you've done so that you are ready for your big race. Rest and recovery is important as well as maintaining race pace work.

TO DO LIST

-
-
-
-
-
-
-

NOTES

-
-
-
-
-
-
-

PHASE 1
BASIC
Building Your Foundation

- Keep running easy, conversational pace, unless it is your speed work.
- Your running week consists of four base runs, one speed day, one long run, and one rest day.

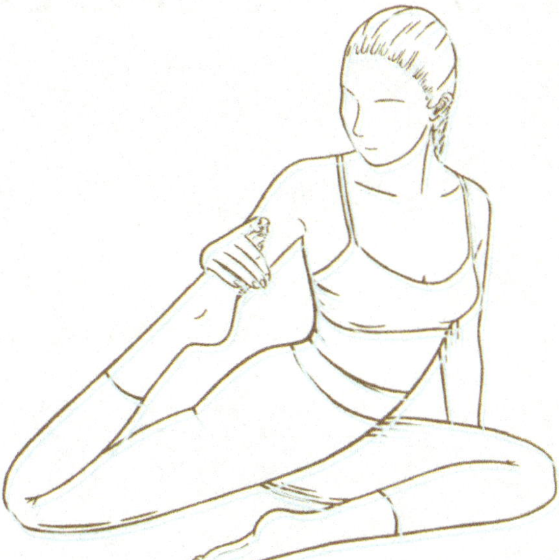

"THE ONLY WAY TO DO GREAT WORK IS TO LOVE WHAT YOU DO."

— STEVE JOBS

The Importance of Your Base Run.

All throughout the year our athletes hear us preach about keeping up with their base runs. Once their race has concluded and recovery has passed (roughly one to two weeks active recovery), it is time to resume your base runs and resume your training, even if you don't have a goal race in mind.

Why Are These Base Runs So Important, and Why Do We Stress Getting These in All Year-Round?

Think of a base run as your running foundation. These runs are part of any distance training plan found from the 5k to the ultra-marathon distance. They are especially important for beginners because, if you think about building a foundation, a beginner will have accumulated less overall lifetime volume than a seasoned runner. If you are new to running, it is important to build a strong aerobic base before you start adding speed-work or other more intense workouts to your training.

How to Perform a Base Run?

A base run is a consistent,`daily run that lasts from 30 minutes to 60 minutes at your perceived relaxed pace (conversational pace, meaning that you should be able to talk in complete sentences without gasping for breath). The distance of your base runs will vary depending on your fitness level and goals. If you are just beginning your running journey, you may start with three mile base runs and gradually increase the distance as you get stronger. Just like your long run, try to increase your base runs 10% about every two to three weeks.

How Long Does it Take to Build Your Base?

It takes about five to six weeks to build a proper base before you start to enter your training phases for an endurance event. Take a moment to think about what a training plan will look like. It begins with a certain amount of mileage and effort. If you jump directly into that plan, there is a very good chance that you either won't be able to complete the workouts or even end up on the injured list. Developing a base will strengthen your musculoskeletal durability. Far too often runners cannot take the demand on their bodies while training for long distances. Running a consistent, easy daily base will help your body adapt. Your legs will grow stronger so you can better handle speed work, long runs, and overall total duration volume, as well as handle any accumulated fatigue in future training.

Running a consistent base will help your body build aerobic efficiency. When you first begin running, your body responds by increasing the number of red blood cells and increasing capillaries in your muscles. The more red blood cells and capillaries you have, the easier it is to transport oxygen throughout your body, the more your body can respond to exercise.

Why Do I Continue Base Runs After My Goal Race?

Imagine you finish your race and then you take the next few months off. All of the foundation that you built up has diminished. When you choose to return to training again, you now have to build your base from the beginning. If you had kept up with your runs, you would most likely return at a place ahead of where you last began and be able to go into your speed, endurance, and harder efforts sooner. This is where you start gradually become a stronger, faster, and more efficient runner over time. When you think about putting in the consistent work year over year that is when you start to see huge gains in your running.

Aerobic v. Anaerobic Training.

Aerobic Capacity Training.

There are two main ways that the body produces energy. One way, includes the use of oxygen, aerobic, meaning "with air." The second way is without the use of oxygen, anaerobic, or "without air." Different percentages of each energy system are used for any exercise depending on duration and intensity. The development of each system should be optimized based on the goal of the individual.

There are several ways to improve aerobic capacity. These generally involve base runs which are done at an easy, or conversational pace, long runs, and lactate threshold runs or intervals. One of the best ways to improve aerobic capacity is to run frequently at the aerobic threshold, or the point at which the body transitions from using fat to glycogen. As an individual gets fitter, the use of fat becomes more efficient and glycogen reserves are saved for higher-intensity work. The aerobic threshold is around 60-75% of maximum heart rate.

The other way to help improve aerobic capacity is to train at the point where the body starts to use lactate as fuel. The intensity just below this point is considered aerobic since the body mostly uses oxygen as energy and creates very few waste products as a result. Just like when training the aerobic threshold, training the lactate threshold improves the ability to use lactate and improves ability to run faster and longer.

Duration & Frequency.

To become a better runner, the amount of time spent running each week is the most important component. It doesn't matter if time or miles are being used to track duration what matters is; that "time on your feet, will help you compete." Running consistently creates adaptations within your musculature system and your nervous system. You are teaching your body to cope with the demands of your training blocks.

Anaerobic Capacity Training.

Anaerobic means "without air." Anaerobic training is about how your body produces energy while utilizing very little oxygen.

This type of training is at high intensity for short bursts, or anything all out under 90 seconds You are pushing out of your usual comfort zone and this should leave you "out of breath." Anaerobic exercise improves, as you adapt to this type of intensity. Examples of this type of training are sprints and speed work. Generally, a lot of recovery time is needed in between reps for the body to properly recover and adapt.

Hills: Hills are a great way to increase leg power and strength. They will help the transition to more formal speed work on the track. When running hills, the runner should focus on their perceived effort and not trying to hit a certain time.

Fartleks: This is a Swedish term meaning "speed play." This can be tailored to the specific event. The proportion of speed can be adjusted to accommodate a more anaerobic vs aerobic focus or vice versa. These are done as a continuous run where varying speed and intensity are changed for different durations throughout the run.

Interval Training: Interval training alternates high-intensity work periods with low-intensity recovery periods. It's an effective way to improve fitness quickly.

PHASE 1

TIP: Base runs should be run at a conversational pace.

WEEK 1: BASIC

DAY 1 Date:	Time: Route:	Mileage: Choice:	: : Y/N
Distance/Time:		Stress/Emotion Tracker ○ ○ ○ ○ ○ VERY SAD ⟷ VERY HAPPY	
Workout:		How did the run feel? ☆ ☆ ☆ ☆ ☆ HARD ⟷ EASY	
Weather:		Water Tracker	
Takeaways:			

DAY 2 Date:	Time: Route:	Mileage: Choice:	: : Y/N
Distance/Time:		Stress/Emotion Tracker ○ ○ ○ ○ ○ VERY SAD ⟷ VERY HAPPY	
Workout:		How did the run feel? ☆ ☆ ☆ ☆ ☆ HARD ⟷ EASY	
Weather:		Water Tracker	
Takeaways:			

DAY 3 Date:	Time: Route:	Mileage: Choice:	: : Y/N
Distance/Time:		Stress/Emotion Tracker ○ ○ ○ ○ ○ VERY SAD ⟷ VERY HAPPY	
Workout:		How did the run feel? ☆ ☆ ☆ ☆ ☆ HARD ⟷ EASY	
Weather:		Water Tracker	
Takeaways:			

DAY 4 Date: | Time: | Route: | Mileage: | Choice: | : | : Y/N

Distance/Time:

Workout:

Weather:

Takeaways:

Stress/Emotion Tracker
○ ○ ○ ○ ○
VERY SAD ⟷ VERY HAPPY

How did the run feel?
☆ ☆ ☆ ☆ ☆
HARD ⟷ EASY

Water Tracker

DAY 5 Date: | Time: | Route: | Mileage: | Choice: | : | : Y/N

Distance/Time:

Workout:

Weather:

Takeaways:

Stress/Emotion Tracker
○ ○ ○ ○ ○
VERY SAD ⟷ VERY HAPPY

How did the run feel?
☆ ☆ ☆ ☆ ☆
HARD ⟷ EASY

Water Tracker

DAY 6 Date: | Time: | Route: | Mileage: | Choice: | : | : Y/N

Distance/Time:

Workout:

Weather:

Takeaways:

Stress/Emotion Tracker
○ ○ ○ ○ ○
VERY SAD ⟷ VERY HAPPY

How did the run feel?
☆ ☆ ☆ ☆ ☆
HARD ⟷ EASY

Water Tracker

DAY 7 Date: | Time: | Route: | Mileage: | Choice: | : | : Y/N

Distance/Time:

Workout:

Weather:

Takeaways:

Stress/Emotion Tracker
○ ○ ○ ○ ○
VERY SAD ⟷ VERY HAPPY

How did the run feel?
☆ ☆ ☆ ☆ ☆
HARD ⟷ EASY

Water Tracker

"SUCCESS IS NOT FINAL, FAILURE IS NOT FATAL: IT IS THE COURAGE TO CONTINUE THAT COUNTS."

— WINSTON CHURCHILL

SELF-CARE Checklist

	M	T	W	TH	F	SA	SU
Drink a glass of water to start the day	☐	☐	☐	☐	☐	☐	☐
Enjoy your run	☐	☐	☐	☐	☐	☐	☐
Get some fresh air	☐	☐	☐	☐	☐	☐	☐
Have a healthy breakfast	☐	☐	☐	☐	☐	☐	☐
Stretch your body	☐	☐	☐	☐	☐	☐	☐
Enjoy your daily mobility	☐	☐	☐	☐	☐	☐	☐
Enjoy some sunshine	☐	☐	☐	☐	☐	☐	☐
Take hot/cold bath or shower	☐	☐	☐	☐	☐	☐	☐
Read something you enjoy	☐	☐	☐	☐	☐	☐	☐
Play some invigorating music	☐	☐	☐	☐	☐	☐	☐
Disconnect	☐	☐	☐	☐	☐	☐	☐
Eat a healthy snack	☐	☐	☐	☐	☐	☐	☐
Wind down by avoiding bright light at night	☐	☐	☐	☐	☐	☐	☐
Get in bed before 10pm	☐	☐	☐	☐	☐	☐	☐

PHASE 1

TIP: Plan your hydration when running 60 minutes or longer - drink three to four sips of water every mile (four ounces every 15 minutes.)

WEEK 2: BASIC

DAY 1	**Time:**	**Mileage:**	:
Date:	**Route:**	**Choice:**	: Y/N

Distance/Time:	**Stress/Emotion Tracker** ○ ○ ○ ○ ○ VERY SAD ⟷ VERY HAPPY
Workout:	**How did the run feel?** ☆ ☆ ☆ ☆ ☆ HARD ⟷ EASY
Weather:	**Water Tracker**
Takeaways:	

DAY 2	**Time:**	**Mileage:**	:
Date:	**Route:**	**Choice:**	: Y/N

Distance/Time:	**Stress/Emotion Tracker** ○ ○ ○ ○ ○ VERY SAD ⟷ VERY HAPPY
Workout:	**How did the run feel?** ☆ ☆ ☆ ☆ ☆ HARD ⟷ EASY
Weather:	**Water Tracker**
Takeaways:	

DAY 3	**Time:**	**Mileage:**	:
Date:	**Route:**	**Choice:**	: Y/N

Distance/Time:	**Stress/Emotion Tracker** ○ ○ ○ ○ ○ VERY SAD ⟷ VERY HAPPY
Workout:	**How did the run feel?** ☆ ☆ ☆ ☆ ☆ HARD ⟷ EASY
Weather:	**Water Tracker**
Takeaways:	

DAY 4	Time:	Mileage:	:
Date:	Route:	Choice:	: Y/N

Distance/Time:	Stress/Emotion Tracker ○ ○ ○ ○ ○ VERY SAD ⟷ VERY HAPPY
Workout:	How did the run feel? ☆ ☆ ☆ ☆ ☆ HARD ⟷ EASY
Weather:	Water Tracker
Takeaways:	

DAY 5	Time:	Mileage:	:
Date:	Route:	Choice:	: Y/N

Distance/Time:	Stress/Emotion Tracker ○ ○ ○ ○ ○ VERY SAD ⟷ VERY HAPPY
Workout:	How did the run feel? ☆ ☆ ☆ ☆ ☆ HARD ⟷ EASY
Weather:	Water Tracker
Takeaways:	

DAY 6	Time:	Mileage:	:
Date:	Route:	Choice:	: Y/N

Distance/Time:	Stress/Emotion Tracker ○ ○ ○ ○ ○ VERY SAD ⟷ VERY HAPPY
Workout:	How did the run feel? ☆ ☆ ☆ ☆ ☆ HARD ⟷ EASY
Weather:	Water Tracker
Takeaways:	

DAY 7	Time:	Mileage:	:
Date:	Route:	Choice:	: Y/N

Distance/Time:	Stress/Emotion Tracker ○ ○ ○ ○ ○ VERY SAD ⟷ VERY HAPPY
Workout:	How did the run feel? ☆ ☆ ☆ ☆ ☆ HARD ⟷ EASY
Weather:	Water Tracker
Takeaways:	

"THE MAN WHO MOVES A MOUNTAIN BEGINS BY CARRYING AWAY SMALL STONES."

— CONFUCIUS

SELF-CARE Checklist

	M	T	W	TH	F	SA	SU
Drink a glass of water to start the day	☐	☐	☐	☐	☐	☐	☐
Enjoy your run	☐	☐	☐	☐	☐	☐	☐
Get some fresh air	☐	☐	☐	☐	☐	☐	☐
Have a healthy breakfast	☐	☐	☐	☐	☐	☐	☐
Stretch your body	☐	☐	☐	☐	☐	☐	☐
Enjoy your daily mobility	☐	☐	☐	☐	☐	☐	☐
Enjoy some sunshine	☐	☐	☐	☐	☐	☐	☐
Take hot/cold bath or shower	☐	☐	☐	☐	☐	☐	☐
Read something you enjoy	☐	☐	☐	☐	☐	☐	☐
Play some invigorating music	☐	☐	☐	☐	☐	☐	☐
Disconnect	☐	☐	☐	☐	☐	☐	☐
Eat a healthy snack	☐	☐	☐	☐	☐	☐	☐
Wind down by avoiding bright light at night	☐	☐	☐	☐	☐	☐	☐
Get in bed before 10pm	☐	☐	☐	☐	☐	☐	☐

PHASE 1

TIP: Grab your foam roller and use for five to ten minutes after a run to release fascial tension.

WEEK 3: BASIC

DAY 1
Date:
Time:
Route:
Mileage:
Choice:
:
: Y/N

Distance/Time:

Workout:

Weather:

Takeaways:

Stress/Emotion Tracker
○ ○ ○ ○ ○
VERY SAD ⟷ VERY HAPPY

How did the run feel?
☆ ☆ ☆ ☆ ☆
HARD ⟷ EASY

Water Tracker

DAY 2
Date:
Time:
Route:
Mileage:
Choice:
:
: Y/N

Distance/Time:

Workout:

Weather:

Takeaways:

Stress/Emotion Tracker
○ ○ ○ ○ ○
VERY SAD ⟷ VERY HAPPY

How did the run feel?
☆ ☆ ☆ ☆ ☆
HARD ⟷ EASY

Water Tracker

DAY 3
Date:
Time:
Route:
Mileage:
Choice:
:
: Y/N

Distance/Time:

Workout:

Weather:

Takeaways:

Stress/Emotion Tracker
○ ○ ○ ○ ○
VERY SAD ⟷ VERY HAPPY

How did the run feel?
☆ ☆ ☆ ☆ ☆
HARD ⟷ EASY

Water Tracker

DAY 4			
Date:	Time:	Mileage:	:
	Route:	Choice:	: Y/N

Distance/Time:

Workout:

Weather:

Takeaways:

Stress/Emotion Tracker

○ ○ ○ ○ ○

VERY SAD ⟷ VERY HAPPY

How did the run feel?

☆ ☆ ☆ ☆ ☆

HARD ⟷ EASY

Water Tracker

DAY 5			
Date:	Time:	Mileage:	:
	Route:	Choice:	: Y/N

Distance/Time:

Workout:

Weather:

Takeaways:

Stress/Emotion Tracker

○ ○ ○ ○ ○

VERY SAD ⟷ VERY HAPPY

How did the run feel?

☆ ☆ ☆ ☆ ☆

HARD ⟷ EASY

Water Tracker

DAY 6			
Date:	Time:	Mileage:	:
	Route:	Choice:	: Y/N

Distance/Time:

Workout:

Weather:

Takeaways:

Stress/Emotion Tracker

○ ○ ○ ○ ○

VERY SAD ⟷ VERY HAPPY

How did the run feel?

☆ ☆ ☆ ☆ ☆

HARD ⟷ EASY

Water Tracker

DAY 7			
Date:	Time:	Mileage:	:
	Route:	Choice:	: Y/N

Distance/Time:

Workout:

Weather:

Takeaways:

Stress/Emotion Tracker

○ ○ ○ ○ ○

VERY SAD ⟷ VERY HAPPY

How did the run feel?

☆ ☆ ☆ ☆ ☆

HARD ⟷ EASY

Water Tracker

"DO NOT WAIT TO STRIKE TILL THE IRON IS HOT; BUT MAKE IT HOT BY STRIKING."

— WILLIAM BUTLER YEATS

SELF-CARE Checklist

	M	T	W	TH	F	SA	SU
Drink a glass of water to start the day	☐	☐	☐	☐	☐	☐	☐
Enjoy your run	☐	☐	☐	☐	☐	☐	☐
Get some fresh air	☐	☐	☐	☐	☐	☐	☐
Have a healthy breakfast	☐	☐	☐	☐	☐	☐	☐
Stretch your body	☐	☐	☐	☐	☐	☐	☐
Enjoy your daily mobility	☐	☐	☐	☐	☐	☐	☐
Enjoy some sunshine	☐	☐	☐	☐	☐	☐	☐
Take hot/cold bath or shower	☐	☐	☐	☐	☐	☐	☐
Read something you enjoy	☐	☐	☐	☐	☐	☐	☐
Play some invigorating music	☐	☐	☐	☐	☐	☐	☐
Disconnect	☐	☐	☐	☐	☐	☐	☐
Eat a healthy snack	☐	☐	☐	☐	☐	☐	☐
Wind down by avoiding bright light at night	☐	☐	☐	☐	☐	☐	☐
Get in bed before 10pm	☐	☐	☐	☐	☐	☐	☐

PHASE 1

TIP: The only bad run is the one you did not do!

WEEK 4: BASIC

DAY 1 Date:	Time: Route:	Mileage: Choice:	: : Y/N
Distance/Time:		Stress/Emotion Tracker ○ ○ ○ ○ ○ VERY SAD ⟷ VERY HAPPY How did the run feel? ☆ ☆ ☆ ☆ ☆ HARD ⟷ EASY Water Tracker	
Workout:			
Weather:			
Takeaways:			

DAY 2 Date:	Time: Route:	Mileage: Choice:	: : Y/N
Distance/Time:		Stress/Emotion Tracker ○ ○ ○ ○ ○ VERY SAD ⟷ VERY HAPPY How did the run feel? ☆ ☆ ☆ ☆ ☆ HARD ⟷ EASY Water Tracker	
Workout:			
Weather:			
Takeaways:			

DAY 3 Date:	Time: Route:	Mileage: Choice:	: : Y/N
Distance/Time:		Stress/Emotion Tracker ○ ○ ○ ○ ○ VERY SAD ⟷ VERY HAPPY How did the run feel? ☆ ☆ ☆ ☆ ☆ HARD ⟷ EASY Water Tracker	
Workout:			
Weather:			
Takeaways:			

DAY 4

Date:

Time:

Route:

Mileage:

Choice:

:

: Y/N

Distance/Time:

Workout:

Weather:

Takeaways:

Stress/Emotion Tracker

○ ○ ○ ○ ○

VERY SAD ⟷ VERY HAPPY

How did the run feel?

☆ ☆ ☆ ☆ ☆

HARD ⟷ EASY

Water Tracker

DAY 5

Date:

Time:

Route:

Mileage:

Choice:

:

: Y/N

Distance/Time:

Workout:

Weather:

Takeaways:

Stress/Emotion Tracker

○ ○ ○ ○ ○

VERY SAD ⟷ VERY HAPPY

How did the run feel?

☆ ☆ ☆ ☆ ☆

HARD ⟷ EASY

Water Tracker

DAY 6

Date:

Time:

Route:

Mileage:

Choice:

:

: Y/N

Distance/Time:

Workout:

Weather:

Takeaways:

Stress/Emotion Tracker

○ ○ ○ ○ ○

VERY SAD ⟷ VERY HAPPY

How did the run feel?

☆ ☆ ☆ ☆ ☆

HARD ⟷ EASY

Water Tracker

DAY 7

Date:

Time:

Route:

Mileage:

Choice:

:

: Y/N

Distance/Time:

Workout:

Weather:

Takeaways:

Stress/Emotion Tracker

○ ○ ○ ○ ○

VERY SAD ⟷ VERY HAPPY

How did the run feel?

☆ ☆ ☆ ☆ ☆

HARD ⟷ EASY

Water Tracker

"IT ALWAYS SEEMS IMPOSSIBLE UNTIL IT'S DONE."

— NELSON MANDELA

SELF-CARE Checklist

	M	T	W	TH	F	SA	SU
Drink a glass of water to start the day	☐	☐	☐	☐	☐	☐	☐
Enjoy your run	☐	☐	☐	☐	☐	☐	☐
Get some fresh air	☐	☐	☐	☐	☐	☐	☐
Have a healthy breakfast	☐	☐	☐	☐	☐	☐	☐
Stretch your body	☐	☐	☐	☐	☐	☐	☐
Enjoy your daily mobility	☐	☐	☐	☐	☐	☐	☐
Enjoy some sunshine	☐	☐	☐	☐	☐	☐	☐
Take hot/cold bath or shower	☐	☐	☐	☐	☐	☐	☐
Read something you enjoy	☐	☐	☐	☐	☐	☐	☐
Play some invigorating music	☐	☐	☐	☐	☐	☐	☐
Disconnect	☐	☐	☐	☐	☐	☐	☐
Eat a healthy snack	☐	☐	☐	☐	☐	☐	☐
Wind down by avoiding bright light at night	☐	☐	☐	☐	☐	☐	☐
Get in bed before 10pm	☐	☐	☐	☐	☐	☐	☐

PHASE 1

TIP: During longer workouts (90+ minutes), your fluid intake should include a sports drink to replenish lost sodium and minerals.

WEEK 5: BASIC

DAY 1 Date:	Time: Route:	Mileage: Choice:	: : Y/N
Distance/Time:			**Stress/Emotion Tracker** ○ ○ ○ ○ ○ VERY SAD ⟷ VERY HAPPY
Workout:			**How did the run feel?** ☆ ☆ ☆ ☆ ☆ HARD ⟷ EASY
Weather:			**Water Tracker**
Takeaways:			

DAY 2 Date:	Time: Route:	Mileage: Choice:	: : Y/N
Distance/Time:			**Stress/Emotion Tracker** ○ ○ ○ ○ ○ VERY SAD ⟷ VERY HAPPY
Workout:			**How did the run feel?** ☆ ☆ ☆ ☆ ☆ HARD ⟷ EASY
Weather:			**Water Tracker**
Takeaways:			

DAY 3 Date:	Time: Route:	Mileage: Choice:	: : Y/N
Distance/Time:			**Stress/Emotion Tracker** ○ ○ ○ ○ ○ VERY SAD ⟷ VERY HAPPY
Workout:			**How did the run feel?** ☆ ☆ ☆ ☆ ☆ HARD ⟷ EASY
Weather:			**Water Tracker**
Takeaways:			

DAY 4	Time:	Mileage:	:
Date:	Route:	Choice:	: Y/N

Distance/Time:	Stress/Emotion Tracker ○ ○ ○ ○ ○ VERY SAD ⟷ VERY HAPPY
Workout:	How did the run feel? ☆ ☆ ☆ ☆ ☆ HARD ⟷ EASY
Weather:	Water Tracker
Takeaways:	

DAY 5	Time:	Mileage:	:
Date:	Route:	Choice:	: Y/N

Distance/Time:	Stress/Emotion Tracker ○ ○ ○ ○ ○ VERY SAD ⟷ VERY HAPPY
Workout:	How did the run feel? ☆ ☆ ☆ ☆ ☆ HARD ⟷ EASY
Weather:	Water Tracker
Takeaways:	

DAY 6	Time:	Mileage:	:
Date:	Route:	Choice:	: Y/N

Distance/Time:	Stress/Emotion Tracker ○ ○ ○ ○ ○ VERY SAD ⟷ VERY HAPPY
Workout:	How did the run feel? ☆ ☆ ☆ ☆ ☆ HARD ⟷ EASY
Weather:	Water Tracker
Takeaways:	

DAY 7	Time:	Mileage:	:
Date:	Route:	Choice:	: Y/N

Distance/Time:	Stress/Emotion Tracker ○ ○ ○ ○ ○ VERY SAD ⟷ VERY HAPPY
Workout:	How did the run feel? ☆ ☆ ☆ ☆ ☆ HARD ⟷ EASY
Weather:	Water Tracker
Takeaways:	

"OUR GREATEST GLORY IS NOT IN NEVER FALLING, BUT IN RISING EVERY TIME WE FALL."

— CONFUCIUS

SELF-CARE *Checklist*

	M	T	W	TH	F	SA	SU
Drink a glass of water to start the day	☐	☐	☐	☐	☐	☐	☐
Enjoy your run	☐	☐	☐	☐	☐	☐	☐
Get some fresh air	☐	☐	☐	☐	☐	☐	☐
Have a healthy breakfast	☐	☐	☐	☐	☐	☐	☐
Stretch your body	☐	☐	☐	☐	☐	☐	☐
Enjoy your daily mobility	☐	☐	☐	☐	☐	☐	☐
Enjoy some sunshine	☐	☐	☐	☐	☐	☐	☐
Take hot/cold bath or shower	☐	☐	☐	☐	☐	☐	☐
Read something you enjoy	☐	☐	☐	☐	☐	☐	☐
Play some invigorating music	☐	☐	☐	☐	☐	☐	☐
Disconnect	☐	☐	☐	☐	☐	☐	☐
Eat a healthy snack	☐	☐	☐	☐	☐	☐	☐
Wind down by avoiding bright light at night	☐	☐	☐	☐	☐	☐	☐
Get in bed before 10pm	☐	☐	☐	☐	☐	☐	☐

Training Notes

Mental Health

Phase 1 Tracker

How was my sleep during the phase?

Approx. hours ____________

Get up time ____________

How was I feeling throughout this phase?

Great Good Okay Not good Awful

Things I am proud of accomplishing

- Base Run
- Speed Session
- Long Run
- Mobility
- Nutirtion
- Rest and Recovery

Other: ____

How am I feeling right now?

Great Good Okay Not good Awful

Am I satisfied with this day?

I am grateful today for

What I like about myself today

What I managed to do today

What I would like to tell myself for tomorrow

Notes

How and what would I like to feel tomorrow

joy appreciation empowered enthusiasm
fun proud strong active love
passion freedom happiness optimism
belief hope inspired courage interest
amusement gratitude delight relaxed
calm confident curious focused
worthy thrilled self-respecting kind

PHASE 2

SPEED

Get Comfortable Running at a Faster Pace

- Practice varying degrees and lengths of speed that will help on race day.
- Introduce your favorite running drills to your warm-up routine.

"THE JOURNEY
OF A THOUSAND
MILES BEGINS
WITH ONE STEP."

— LAO TZU

Why a Distance Runner Needs Speed Sessions.

Why would a distance runner do speed workouts, isn't that for sprinters? Isn't that for more serious athletes? Won't going fast injure me? I will never be a fast runner, why should I even do it? These are some of the questions coaches get when it comes to speed workouts; however, it IS true that an athlete should be incorporating a quality speed workout once to twice a week. As a distance runner, you typically have four days of easy, base runs; your long run; and one day of QUALITY - speed workouts.

So, Why Would a Distance Runner Incorporate These into the Routine?

Speed workouts, quite simply, help you become a better runner. By running at a faster pace, you increase ground reaction force (the force exerted by the ground on a body coming into contact with it), improve on running economy, and improve on agility/flexibility, while also reducing the likelihood of injury. The more efficiently you run, the less likely you will become injured.

> "As a Division 1 collegiate sprinter at Virginia Tech I was always aware of how important speed drills are in making me an overall faster runner, and it was pretty obvious that speed was what I needed as a sprinter. At the time, what I didn't realize was how the speed drills that I was doing as a sprinter would years later also make me a more efficient and faster distance runner."
> - Ilmani Mack, Physical Therapist (from The Importance of Speed Workouts for Distance Runners)

What Happens to Your Body When You Perform

These Speed Workouts That Will Transfer to Helping Your Overall Fitness?

During speed workouts you activate your slow-twitch muscles and intermediate muscle fibers. This increases your aerobic capacity.

Myoglobin is a protein found in your muscles and speed workouts increase the production of this protein. Why would you want to increase this protein? Because myoglobin transports oxygen to the mitochondria in your muscles.

Mitochondria produce ATP (energy). By increasing your myoglobin, you improve your body's ability to quickly transport oxygen to the muscles for energy, making you able to run faster.

Increase Your V02Max.

Your VO2max is somewhat limited by your genetics; however, you will see many benefits from performing continued speed-work, especially workouts that target improving your V02Max. When you see improvements in V02Max, your body will become more efficient at recruiting your fast-twitch muscles. Your running economy improves, so that you expend less energy and can run faster at the same effort level. In addition, your ability to tolerate and clear lactic acid improves which helps you sustain a faster pace for longer.

Practicing a Skill.

There is the skill aspect to running. In order to get better at a certain skill, there needs to be variation. So by practicing different ranges of paces from sprinting to easy long runs, you will become a better runner. If you want to run faster, you have to practice running faster! You also need to practice running slower. Speed workouts train you how to output more effort, maintain a higher cadence, and mentally cope with some physical discomfort while running. If you practice this skill once or twice per week consistently, you won't just become faster - you will run faster with less effort.

Are You Intimidated by Doing Full-Blown Speed Sessions?

Improvements in running economy and everything that was mentioned above isn't limited to doing only speed sessions. If you are looking to make improvements in your running, but aren't quite ready, or want additional improvements without the fatigue, use strides to practice running quickly. Strides aren't all out, but they will help to reinforce faster running and recruitment of fast twitch muscles fibers. You may not see benefits right away, but when done consistently you will notice improvements in your running.
(adapted from www.runkeeper.com)

Aim Lower.

It is often times celebrated when one completely goes above and beyond and gives "110% of themselves 120% of the time." More often than not in running, the very opposite is necessary for performance gains and growth. This is because adaptations can occur over a range of a certain stimulus and within that range the benefits you receive from hitting on the high range of your target are the same (or basically the same) as hitting your low range of your target.

When a workout is given by a coach, they are aiming to get the athlete to hit a certain percentage of effort for a duration of time/distance in order to elicit a specific adaptation. If that range isn't hit, then the intended adaptation won't occur as effectively as it would if it did.

What athletes sometimes forget is that hitting the low (read slower) end of the range will satisfy the adaption just as effectively as the upper (read faster) end of the range. Athletes even more so forget that hitting out of range (read much faster) than the target effort will yield either the same benefit or in some cases have negative impact on adaptation. This can lead to slower recovery times, over-training, etc. When an athlete goes harder than prescribed, they are stressing the body too much either mechanically or chemically which leads to faster or more breakdown in the short and long term.

For example: Running easy runs too hard. A lot of times, runners will run too hard on their easy days, whether it be from meeting a friend who is a little faster or naturally on their own. Many of us believe that a run is not complete unless a feeling of complete exhaustion comes upon us. We feel that we did not put in enough "work."

This, however, could not be further from the truth. The main goal of an easy run is to run...easy. This helps to support recovery and build an aerobic base which is essential for endurance running. Running at a higher intensity more often than not can lead to unnecessary stress and fatigue which can ultimately lead to lack of motivation and even injury.

So, how do you know how often and what effort level you should be running? It depends. What are your goals? What distance/time piques your interest? What do you want to get out of running? How much time (daily and throughout the year) do you have available to give to running? With these questions answered there are many groups/coaches/forums that can help guide your way so that when you set out to go for a run or workout, you know what the intent is and how to manage your effort throughout. You will also know where the workout fits in the grand scheme of your training.

Ultimately, whether you decide to join a group, have a personalized coach, or self-coach, remembering to aim lower will help set you up better for growth and consistency for a long career. Everyone is always looking for easy and efficient hacks and this can be considered one of them.

If you have more interest in personalized running coaching and getting the most out of yourself please take a look at our running services at https://www.milesandmacros.net/individual-training or scanning the QR code below.

PHASE 2

TIP: Give yourself periodic "rest weeks" by dropping your mileage every fourth week.

WEEK 6: SPEED

DAY 1	Time:	Mileage:	:
Date:	Route:	Choice:	: Y/N

Distance/Time:	Stress/Emotion Tracker ○ ○ ○ ○ ○ VERY SAD ⟷ VERY HAPPY
Workout:	How did the run feel? ☆ ☆ ☆ ☆ ☆ HARD ⟷ EASY
Weather:	Water Tracker
Takeaways:	

DAY 2	Time:	Mileage:	:
Date:	Route:	Choice:	: Y/N

Distance/Time:	Stress/Emotion Tracker ○ ○ ○ ○ ○ VERY SAD ⟷ VERY HAPPY
Workout:	How did the run feel? ☆ ☆ ☆ ☆ ☆ HARD ⟷ EASY
Weather:	Water Tracker
Takeaways:	

DAY 3	Time:	Mileage:	:
Date:	Route:	Choice:	: Y/N

Distance/Time:	Stress/Emotion Tracker ○ ○ ○ ○ ○ VERY SAD ⟷ VERY HAPPY
Workout:	How did the run feel? ☆ ☆ ☆ ☆ ☆ HARD ⟷ EASY
Weather:	Water Tracker
Takeaways:	

DAY 4
Date:
Time:
Route:
Mileage:
Choice:
:
: Y/N

Distance/Time:
Workout:
Weather:
Takeaways:

Stress/Emotion Tracker
○ ○ ○ ○ ○
VERY SAD ⟷ VERY HAPPY
How did the run feel?
☆ ☆ ☆ ☆ ☆
HARD ⟷ EASY
Water Tracker

DAY 5
Date:
Time:
Route:
Mileage:
Choice:
:
: Y/N

Distance/Time:
Workout:
Weather:
Takeaways:

Stress/Emotion Tracker
○ ○ ○ ○ ○
VERY SAD ⟷ VERY HAPPY
How did the run feel?
☆ ☆ ☆ ☆ ☆
HARD ⟷ EASY
Water Tracker

DAY 6
Date:
Time:
Route:
Mileage:
Choice:
:
: Y/N

Distance/Time:
Workout:
Weather:
Takeaways:

Stress/Emotion Tracker
○ ○ ○ ○ ○
VERY SAD ⟷ VERY HAPPY
How did the run feel?
☆ ☆ ☆ ☆ ☆
HARD ⟷ EASY
Water Tracker

DAY 7
Date:
Time:
Route:
Mileage:
Choice:
:
: Y/N

Distance/Time:
Workout:
Weather:
Takeaways:

Stress/Emotion Tracker
○ ○ ○ ○ ○
VERY SAD ⟷ VERY HAPPY
How did the run feel?
☆ ☆ ☆ ☆ ☆
HARD ⟷ EASY
Water Tracker

"DON'T WATCH THE CLOCK; DO WHAT IT DOES. KEEP GOING."

— SAM LEVENSON

SELF-CARE Checklist

	M	T	W	TH	F	SA	SU
Drink a glass of water to start the day	☐	☐	☐	☐	☐	☐	☐
Enjoy your run	☐	☐	☐	☐	☐	☐	☐
Get some fresh air	☐	☐	☐	☐	☐	☐	☐
Have a healthy breakfast	☐	☐	☐	☐	☐	☐	☐
Stretch your body	☐	☐	☐	☐	☐	☐	☐
Enjoy your daily mobility	☐	☐	☐	☐	☐	☐	☐
Enjoy some sunshine	☐	☐	☐	☐	☐	☐	☐
Take hot/cold bath or shower	☐	☐	☐	☐	☐	☐	☐
Read something you enjoy	☐	☐	☐	☐	☐	☐	☐
Play some invigorating music	☐	☐	☐	☐	☐	☐	☐
Disconnect	☐	☐	☐	☐	☐	☐	☐
Eat a healthy snack	☐	☐	☐	☐	☐	☐	☐
Wind down by avoiding bright light at night	☐	☐	☐	☐	☐	☐	☐
Get in bed before 10pm	☐	☐	☐	☐	☐	☐	☐

PHASE 2

TIP: The introduction of running drills can reinforce the most fundamental concepts behind running performance.

WEEK 7: SPEED

DAY 1 Date:	Time: Route:	Mileage: Choice:	: : Y/N
Distance/Time:		Stress/Emotion Tracker ○ ○ ○ ○ ○ VERY SAD ⟷ VERY HAPPY	
Workout:		How did the run feel? ☆ ☆ ☆ ☆ ☆ HARD ⟷ EASY	
Weather:		Water Tracker	
Takeaways:			

DAY 2 Date:	Time: Route:	Mileage: Choice:	: : Y/N
Distance/Time:		Stress/Emotion Tracker ○ ○ ○ ○ ○ VERY SAD ⟷ VERY HAPPY	
Workout:		How did the run feel? ☆ ☆ ☆ ☆ ☆ HARD ⟷ EASY	
Weather:		Water Tracker	
Takeaways:			

DAY 3 Date:	Time: Route:	Mileage: Choice:	: : Y/N
Distance/Time:		Stress/Emotion Tracker ○ ○ ○ ○ ○ VERY SAD ⟷ VERY HAPPY	
Workout:		How did the run feel? ☆ ☆ ☆ ☆ ☆ HARD ⟷ EASY	
Weather:		Water Tracker	
Takeaways:			

DAY 4
Date:
Time:
Route:
Mileage:
Choice:
:
: Y/N

Distance/Time:
Workout:
Weather:
Takeaways:

Stress/Emotion Tracker
○ ○ ○ ○ ○
VERY SAD ⟷ VERY HAPPY
How did the run feel?
☆ ☆ ☆ ☆ ☆
HARD ⟷ EASY
Water Tracker

DAY 5
Date:
Time:
Route:
Mileage:
Choice:
:
: Y/N

Distance/Time:
Workout:
Weather:
Takeaways:

Stress/Emotion Tracker
○ ○ ○ ○ ○
VERY SAD ⟷ VERY HAPPY
How did the run feel?
☆ ☆ ☆ ☆ ☆
HARD ⟷ EASY
Water Tracker

DAY 6
Date:
Time:
Route:
Mileage:
Choice:
:
: Y/N

Distance/Time:
Workout:
Weather:
Takeaways:

Stress/Emotion Tracker
○ ○ ○ ○ ○
VERY SAD ⟷ VERY HAPPY
How did the run feel?
☆ ☆ ☆ ☆ ☆
HARD ⟷ EASY
Water Tracker

DAY 7
Date:
Time:
Route:
Mileage:
Choice:
:
: Y/N

Distance/Time:
Workout:
Weather:
Takeaways:

Stress/Emotion Tracker
○ ○ ○ ○ ○
VERY SAD ⟷ VERY HAPPY
How did the run feel?
☆ ☆ ☆ ☆ ☆
HARD ⟷ EASY
Water Tracker

"WHAT LIES BEHIND US AND WHAT LIES BEFORE US ARE TINY MATTERS COMPARED TO WHAT LIES WITHIN US."

— RALPH WALDO EMERSON

SELF-CARE Checklist

	M	T	W	TH	F	SA	SU
Drink a glass of water to start the day	☐	☐	☐	☐	☐	☐	☐
Enjoy your run	☐	☐	☐	☐	☐	☐	☐
Get some fresh air	☐	☐	☐	☐	☐	☐	☐
Have a healthy breakfast	☐	☐	☐	☐	☐	☐	☐
Stretch your body	☐	☐	☐	☐	☐	☐	☐
Enjoy your daily mobility	☐	☐	☐	☐	☐	☐	☐
Enjoy some sunshine	☐	☐	☐	☐	☐	☐	☐
Take hot/cold bath or shower	☐	☐	☐	☐	☐	☐	☐
Read something you enjoy	☐	☐	☐	☐	☐	☐	☐
Play some invigorating music	☐	☐	☐	☐	☐	☐	☐
Disconnect	☐	☐	☐	☐	☐	☐	☐
Eat a healthy snack	☐	☐	☐	☐	☐	☐	☐
Wind down by avoiding bright light at night	☐	☐	☐	☐	☐	☐	☐
Get in bed before 10pm	☐	☐	☐	☐	☐	☐	☐

PHASE 2

TIP: Fueling needs to be introduced early into your training block. Get used to taking in calories on your long runs.

WEEK 8: SPEED

DAY 1
Date:
Time:
Route:
Mileage:
Choice:
:
: Y/N

Distance/Time:
Workout:
Weather:
Takeaways:

Stress/Emotion Tracker
○ ○ ○ ○ ○
VERY SAD ⟷ VERY HAPPY
How did the run feel?
☆ ☆ ☆ ☆ ☆
HARD ⟷ EASY
Water Tracker

DAY 2
Date:
Time:
Route:
Mileage:
Choice:
:
: Y/N

Distance/Time:
Workout:
Weather:
Takeaways:

Stress/Emotion Tracker
○ ○ ○ ○ ○
VERY SAD ⟷ VERY HAPPY
How did the run feel?
☆ ☆ ☆ ☆ ☆
HARD ⟷ EASY
Water Tracker

DAY 3
Date:
Time:
Route:
Mileage:
Choice:
:
: Y/N

Distance/Time:
Workout:
Weather:
Takeaways:

Stress/Emotion Tracker
○ ○ ○ ○ ○
VERY SAD ⟷ VERY HAPPY
How did the run feel?
☆ ☆ ☆ ☆ ☆
HARD ⟷ EASY
Water Tracker

DAY 4 Date: | Time: Route: | Mileage: Choice: | : | : Y/N

Distance/Time:

Workout:

Weather:

Takeaways:

Stress/Emotion Tracker
○ ○ ○ ○ ○
VERY SAD ⟷ VERY HAPPY
How did the run feel?
☆ ☆ ☆ ☆ ☆
HARD ⟷ EASY
Water Tracker

DAY 5 Date: | Time: Route: | Mileage: Choice: | : | : Y/N

Distance/Time:

Workout:

Weather:

Takeaways:

Stress/Emotion Tracker
○ ○ ○ ○ ○
VERY SAD ⟷ VERY HAPPY
How did the run feel?
☆ ☆ ☆ ☆ ☆
HARD ⟷ EASY
Water Tracker

DAY 6 Date: | Time: Route: | Mileage: Choice: | : | : Y/N

Distance/Time:

Workout:

Weather:

Takeaways:

Stress/Emotion Tracker
○ ○ ○ ○ ○
VERY SAD ⟷ VERY HAPPY
How did the run feel?
☆ ☆ ☆ ☆ ☆
HARD ⟷ EASY
Water Tracker

DAY 7 Date: | Time: Route: | Mileage: Choice: | : | : Y/N

Distance/Time:

Workout:

Weather:

Takeaways:

Stress/Emotion Tracker
○ ○ ○ ○ ○
VERY SAD ⟷ VERY HAPPY
How did the run feel?
☆ ☆ ☆ ☆ ☆
HARD ⟷ EASY
Water Tracker

"BELIEVE YOU CAN AND YOU'RE HALFWAY THERE."

— THEODORE ROOSEVELT

SELF-CARE Checklist

	M	T	W	TH	F	SA	SU
Drink a glass of water to start the day	☐	☐	☐	☐	☐	☐	☐
Enjoy your run	☐	☐	☐	☐	☐	☐	☐
Get some fresh air	☐	☐	☐	☐	☐	☐	☐
Have a healthy breakfast	☐	☐	☐	☐	☐	☐	☐
Stretch your body	☐	☐	☐	☐	☐	☐	☐
Enjoy your daily mobility	☐	☐	☐	☐	☐	☐	☐
Enjoy some sunshine	☐	☐	☐	☐	☐	☐	☐
Take hot/cold bath or shower	☐	☐	☐	☐	☐	☐	☐
Read something you enjoy	☐	☐	☐	☐	☐	☐	☐
Play some invigorating music	☐	☐	☐	☐	☐	☐	☐
Disconnect	☐	☐	☐	☐	☐	☐	☐
Eat a healthy snack	☐	☐	☐	☐	☐	☐	☐
Wind down by avoiding bright light at night	☐	☐	☐	☐	☐	☐	☐
Get in bed before 10pm	☐	☐	☐	☐	☐	☐	☐

PHASE 2

TIP: Practice with what you plan to use on race-day. NEVER try anything new on race-day!

WEEK 9: SPEED

DAY 1
Date: | Time: | Route: | Mileage: | Choice: | : | : Y/N

Distance/Time:

Workout:

Weather:

Takeaways:

Stress/Emotion Tracker
○ ○ ○ ○ ○
VERY SAD ⟷ VERY HAPPY

How did the run feel?
☆ ☆ ☆ ☆ ☆
HARD ⟷ EASY

Water Tracker

DAY 2
Date: | Time: | Route: | Mileage: | Choice: | : | : Y/N

Distance/Time:

Workout:

Weather:

Takeaways:

Stress/Emotion Tracker
○ ○ ○ ○ ○
VERY SAD ⟷ VERY HAPPY

How did the run feel?
☆ ☆ ☆ ☆ ☆
HARD ⟷ EASY

Water Tracker

DAY 3
Date: | Time: | Route: | Mileage: | Choice: | : | : Y/N

Distance/Time:

Workout:

Weather:

Takeaways:

Stress/Emotion Tracker
○ ○ ○ ○ ○
VERY SAD ⟷ VERY HAPPY

How did the run feel?
☆ ☆ ☆ ☆ ☆
HARD ⟷ EASY

Water Tracker

DAY 4
Date:
Time:
Route:
Mileage:
Choice:
:
: Y/N

Distance/Time:

Workout:

Weather:

Takeaways:

Stress/Emotion Tracker
○ ○ ○ ○ ○
VERY SAD ⟷ VERY HAPPY
How did the run feel?
☆ ☆ ☆ ☆ ☆
HARD ⟷ EASY
Water Tracker

DAY 5
Date:
Time:
Route:
Mileage:
Choice:
:
: Y/N

Distance/Time:

Workout:

Weather:

Takeaways:

Stress/Emotion Tracker
○ ○ ○ ○ ○
VERY SAD ⟷ VERY HAPPY
How did the run feel?
☆ ☆ ☆ ☆ ☆
HARD ⟷ EASY
Water Tracker

DAY 6
Date:
Time:
Route:
Mileage:
Choice:
:
: Y/N

Distance/Time:

Workout:

Weather:

Takeaways:

Stress/Emotion Tracker
○ ○ ○ ○ ○
VERY SAD ⟷ VERY HAPPY
How did the run feel?
☆ ☆ ☆ ☆ ☆
HARD ⟷ EASY
Water Tracker

DAY 7
Date:
Time:
Route:
Mileage:
Choice:
:
: Y/N

Distance/Time:

Workout:

Weather:

Takeaways:

Stress/Emotion Tracker
○ ○ ○ ○ ○
VERY SAD ⟷ VERY HAPPY
How did the run feel?
☆ ☆ ☆ ☆ ☆
HARD ⟷ EASY
Water Tracker

"HE WHO IS NOT COURAGEOUS ENOUGH TO TAKE RISKS WILL ACCOMPLISH NOTHING IN LIFE."

— MUHAMMAD ALI

SELF-CARE Checklist

	M	T	W	TH	F	SA	SU
Drink a glass of water to start the day	☐	☐	☐	☐	☐	☐	☐
Enjoy your run	☐	☐	☐	☐	☐	☐	☐
Get some fresh air	☐	☐	☐	☐	☐	☐	☐
Have a healthy breakfast	☐	☐	☐	☐	☐	☐	☐
Stretch your body	☐	☐	☐	☐	☐	☐	☐
Enjoy your daily mobility	☐	☐	☐	☐	☐	☐	☐
Enjoy some sunshine	☐	☐	☐	☐	☐	☐	☐
Take hot/cold bath or shower	☐	☐	☐	☐	☐	☐	☐
Read something you enjoy	☐	☐	☐	☐	☐	☐	☐
Play some invigorating music	☐	☐	☐	☐	☐	☐	☐
Disconnect	☐	☐	☐	☐	☐	☐	☐
Eat a healthy snack	☐	☐	☐	☐	☐	☐	☐
Wind down by avoiding bright light at night	☐	☐	☐	☐	☐	☐	☐
Get in bed before 10pm	☐	☐	☐	☐	☐	☐	☐

Training Notes

Mental Health

Phase 2 Tracker

How was my sleep during the phase?

Approx. hours ____________

Get up time ____________

How was I feeling throughout this phase?

Great Good Okay Not good Awful

Things I am proud of accomplishing

- Base Run
- Speed Session
- Long Run
- Mobility
- Nutirtion
- Rest and Recovery

Other: ____________

How am I feeling right now?

Great Good Okay Not good Awful

Am I satisfied with this day?

I am grateful today for

What I like about myself today

What I managed to do today

What I would like to tell myself for tomorrow

Notes

How and what would I like to feel tomorrow

joy appreciation empowered enthusiasm
fun proud strong active love
passion freedom happiness optimism
belief hope inspired courage interest
amusement gratitude delight relaxed
calm confident curious focused
worthy thrilled self-respecting kind

PHASE 3

SPECIFIC

Mimic Your Race-Day Demands

- Practice your race pace.
- Practice on the terrain you will be racing on.
- Think about your elevation gain.

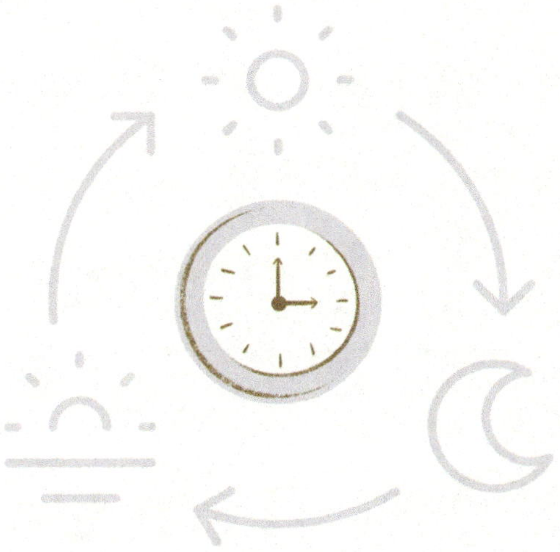

"STRENGTH DOES NOT COME FROM PHYSICAL CAPACITY. IT COMES FROM AN INDOMITABLE WILL."

— MAHATMA GANDHI

How to Implement Specific Training for Your Race-Day.

Racing season seems to approach quickly and it is not always easy to feel a sense of rejuvenation that comes with the season. BUT NOT SO FAST! Don't get too confident with your winter aerobic fitness and strength gains. Remember to take into consideration all that goes into racing. Below is a list of pointers that you can use to ensure that you are as well-prepared as possible for race-day!

Know Your Course and Practice For It.

Understand the course profile, and know that the little lines moving up and down don't account for everything (a small looking bump at mile 25 in your marathon may feel like climbing Mt. Everest)! Look at the number of turns (switchbacks, if on the trail) which can throw off your momentum, get an idea of the terrain, look at past results or ask a friend who has done the course to get an idea of what your finishing time may be. Is your course all (or mostly) downhill? Practicing downhills will help prepare you for the muscular fatigue that you will experience on race-day. What is the typical weather (and even worst case) to know if you need to start to acclimatize your body and mentally prepare for the heat, cold, dryness, or humidity.

Practice in Your Race-Day Kit.

Even though a lot of shoes today have minimal break in periods, it's still best to have run in them before race-day. I typically like putting in at least 50 to 100 miles on them before race-day. Will there be any required gear either at the start due to weather (cold mornings) or mandated by the race? Do you need a drop bag or change of clothes? Know this and make sure you have it all prepared ahead of time so you are not rushing race week or day.

Race-Day Nutrition.

Dial in your race-day nutrition. Being knowledgeable about how many aid stations there are and what they provide on course, the distance between stations, and what that means for how much you need to have on you in terms of cal/hr will be key in execution. Nutrition can become complicated especially when race-day conditions can vary from training conditions. Having a general plan and being flexible with where your energy comes from, as well as your water and electrolyte intake, can be important to race-day success.

Race-Day Hype and Environment.

It is good to know the atmosphere you are entering for race weekend and where you get your energy from. If you signed up for a large marathon, know that there will be a lot of people, large crowds, and carve yourself time for re-energizing, if you are someone who needs it. It can be easy to get caught up in the race-day excitement no matter who you are and you will have extra energy from tapering, but don't waste it in the day(s) before.

Summary.

There are many ways to prepare yourself for success. Knowing and understanding what could happen on race-day will help you be ready for success no matter if things don't go to plan. Going through the physical and mental preparation beforehand makes smaller decisions or adjustments on race-day that much easier.

PHASE 3

TIP: Including a few strides at the end of your base runs can boost your running economy.

WEEK 10: SPECIFIC

DAY 1
Date:
Time:
Route:
Mileage:
Choice:
:
: Y/N

Distance/Time:
Workout:
Weather:
Takeaways:

Stress/Emotion Tracker
○ ○ ○ ○ ○
VERY SAD ⟷ VERY HAPPY
How did the run feel?
☆ ☆ ☆ ☆ ☆
HARD ⟷ EASY
Water Tracker

DAY 2
Date:
Time:
Route:
Mileage:
Choice:
:
: Y/N

Distance/Time:
Workout:
Weather:
Takeaways:

Stress/Emotion Tracker
○ ○ ○ ○ ○
VERY SAD ⟷ VERY HAPPY
How did the run feel?
☆ ☆ ☆ ☆ ☆
HARD ⟷ EASY
Water Tracker

DAY 3
Date:
Time:
Route:
Mileage:
Choice:
:
: Y/N

Distance/Time:
Workout:
Weather:
Takeaways:

Stress/Emotion Tracker
○ ○ ○ ○ ○
VERY SAD ⟷ VERY HAPPY
How did the run feel?
☆ ☆ ☆ ☆ ☆
HARD ⟷ EASY
Water Tracker

DAY 4 Time: Mileage: :
Date: Route: Choice: : Y/N

Distance/Time:
Workout:
Weather:
Takeaways:

Stress/Emotion Tracker
○ ○ ○ ○ ○
VERY SAD ⟷ VERY HAPPY
How did the run feel?
☆ ☆ ☆ ☆ ☆
HARD ⟷ EASY
Water Tracker

DAY 5 Time: Mileage: :
Date: Route: Choice: : Y/N

Distance/Time:
Workout:
Weather:
Takeaways:

Stress/Emotion Tracker
○ ○ ○ ○ ○
VERY SAD ⟷ VERY HAPPY
How did the run feel?
☆ ☆ ☆ ☆ ☆
HARD ⟷ EASY
Water Tracker

DAY 6 Time: Mileage: :
Date: Route: Choice: : Y/N

Distance/Time:
Workout:
Weather:
Takeaways:

Stress/Emotion Tracker
○ ○ ○ ○ ○
VERY SAD ⟷ VERY HAPPY
How did the run feel?
☆ ☆ ☆ ☆ ☆
HARD ⟷ EASY
Water Tracker

DAY 7 Time: Mileage: :
Date: Route: Choice: : Y/N

Distance/Time:
Workout:
Weather:
Takeaways:

Stress/Emotion Tracker
○ ○ ○ ○ ○
VERY SAD ⟷ VERY HAPPY
How did the run feel?
☆ ☆ ☆ ☆ ☆
HARD ⟷ EASY
Water Tracker

"YOU MISS 100% OF THE SHOTS YOU DON'T TAKE."

— WAYNE GRETZKY

SELF-CARE Checklist

	M	T	W	TH	F	SA	SU
Drink a glass of water to start the day	☐	☐	☐	☐	☐	☐	☐
Enjoy your run	☐	☐	☐	☐	☐	☐	☐
Get some fresh air	☐	☐	☐	☐	☐	☐	☐
Have a healthy breakfast	☐	☐	☐	☐	☐	☐	☐
Stretch your body	☐	☐	☐	☐	☐	☐	☐
Enjoy your daily mobility	☐	☐	☐	☐	☐	☐	☐
Enjoy some sunshine	☐	☐	☐	☐	☐	☐	☐
Take hot/cold bath or shower	☐	☐	☐	☐	☐	☐	☐
Read something you enjoy	☐	☐	☐	☐	☐	☐	☐
Play some invigorating music	☐	☐	☐	☐	☐	☐	☐
Disconnect	☐	☐	☐	☐	☐	☐	☐
Eat a healthy snack	☐	☐	☐	☐	☐	☐	☐
Wind down by avoiding bright light at night	☐	☐	☐	☐	☐	☐	☐
Get in bed before 10pm	☐	☐	☐	☐	☐	☐	☐

PHASE 3

TIP: Bodies rely on glycogen as its primary fuel source. Glycogen comes from eating carbohydrates and is stored in the muscles and liver for easily accessible energy.

WEEK 11: SPECIFIC

DAY 1 Date: | Time: Route: | Mileage: Choice: | : : Y/N

Distance/Time:

Workout:

Weather:

Takeaways:

Stress/Emotion Tracker
○ ○ ○ ○ ○
VERY SAD ⟷ VERY HAPPY

How did the run feel?
☆ ☆ ☆ ☆ ☆
HARD ⟷ EASY

Water Tracker

DAY 2 Date: | Time: Route: | Mileage: Choice: | : : Y/N

Distance/Time:

Workout:

Weather:

Takeaways:

Stress/Emotion Tracker
○ ○ ○ ○ ○
VERY SAD ⟷ VERY HAPPY

How did the run feel?
☆ ☆ ☆ ☆ ☆
HARD ⟷ EASY

Water Tracker

DAY 3 Date: | Time: Route: | Mileage: Choice: | : : Y/N

Distance/Time:

Workout:

Weather:

Takeaways:

Stress/Emotion Tracker
○ ○ ○ ○ ○
VERY SAD ⟷ VERY HAPPY

How did the run feel?
☆ ☆ ☆ ☆ ☆
HARD ⟷ EASY

Water Tracker

DAY 4	Time:	Mileage:	:
Date:	Route:	Choice:	: Y/N

Distance/Time:	Stress/Emotion Tracker ○ ○ ○ ○ ○ VERY SAD ⟷ VERY HAPPY
Workout:	How did the run feel? ☆ ☆ ☆ ☆ ☆ HARD ⟷ EASY
Weather:	Water Tracker
Takeaways:	

DAY 5	Time:	Mileage:	:
Date:	Route:	Choice:	: Y/N

Distance/Time:	Stress/Emotion Tracker ○ ○ ○ ○ ○ VERY SAD ⟷ VERY HAPPY
Workout:	How did the run feel? ☆ ☆ ☆ ☆ ☆ HARD ⟷ EASY
Weather:	Water Tracker
Takeaways:	

DAY 6	Time:	Mileage:	:
Date:	Route:	Choice:	: Y/N

Distance/Time:	Stress/Emotion Tracker ○ ○ ○ ○ ○ VERY SAD ⟷ VERY HAPPY
Workout:	How did the run feel? ☆ ☆ ☆ ☆ ☆ HARD ⟷ EASY
Weather:	Water Tracker
Takeaways:	

DAY 7	Time:	Mileage:	:
Date:	Route:	Choice:	: Y/N

Distance/Time:	Stress/Emotion Tracker ○ ○ ○ ○ ○ VERY SAD ⟷ VERY HAPPY
Workout:	How did the run feel? ☆ ☆ ☆ ☆ ☆ HARD ⟷ EASY
Weather:	Water Tracker
Takeaways:	

"PAIN IS TEMPORARY. QUITTING LASTS FOREVER."

— LANCE ARMSTRONG

SELF-CARE Checklist

	M	T	W	TH	F	SA	SU
Drink a glass of water to start the day	☐	☐	☐	☐	☐	☐	☐
Enjoy your run	☐	☐	☐	☐	☐	☐	☐
Get some fresh air	☐	☐	☐	☐	☐	☐	☐
Have a healthy breakfast	☐	☐	☐	☐	☐	☐	☐
Stretch your body	☐	☐	☐	☐	☐	☐	☐
Enjoy your daily mobility	☐	☐	☐	☐	☐	☐	☐
Enjoy some sunshine	☐	☐	☐	☐	☐	☐	☐
Take hot/cold bath or shower	☐	☐	☐	☐	☐	☐	☐
Read something you enjoy	☐	☐	☐	☐	☐	☐	☐
Play some invigorating music	☐	☐	☐	☐	☐	☐	☐
Disconnect	☐	☐	☐	☐	☐	☐	☐
Eat a healthy snack	☐	☐	☐	☐	☐	☐	☐
Wind down by avoiding bright light at night	☐	☐	☐	☐	☐	☐	☐
Get in bed before 10pm	☐	☐	☐	☐	☐	☐	☐

PHASE 3

TIP: Post-injury rehab and recovery can require up to an additional 20% more calories.

WEEK 12: SPECIFIC

DAY 1
Date:
Time:
Route:
Mileage:
Choice:
:
: Y/N

Distance/Time:

Workout:

Weather:

Takeaways:

Stress/Emotion Tracker
○ ○ ○ ○ ○
VERY SAD ⟷ VERY HAPPY

How did the run feel?
☆ ☆ ☆ ☆ ☆
HARD ⟷ EASY

Water Tracker

DAY 2
Date:
Time:
Route:
Mileage:
Choice:
:
: Y/N

Distance/Time:

Workout:

Weather:

Takeaways:

Stress/Emotion Tracker
○ ○ ○ ○ ○
VERY SAD ⟷ VERY HAPPY

How did the run feel?
☆ ☆ ☆ ☆ ☆
HARD ⟷ EASY

Water Tracker

DAY 3
Date:
Time:
Route:
Mileage:
Choice:
:
: Y/N

Distance/Time:

Workout:

Weather:

Takeaways:

Stress/Emotion Tracker
○ ○ ○ ○ ○
VERY SAD ⟷ VERY HAPPY

How did the run feel?
☆ ☆ ☆ ☆ ☆
HARD ⟷ EASY

Water Tracker

DAY 4 Time: Mileage: :
Date: Route: Choice: : Y/N

Distance/Time:
Workout:
Weather:
Takeaways:

Stress/Emotion Tracker
○ ○ ○ ○ ○
VERY SAD ⟷ VERY HAPPY
How did the run feel?
☆ ☆ ☆ ☆ ☆
HARD ⟷ EASY
Water Tracker

DAY 5 Time: Mileage: :
Date: Route: Choice: : Y/N

Distance/Time:
Workout:
Weather:
Takeaways:

Stress/Emotion Tracker
○ ○ ○ ○ ○
VERY SAD ⟷ VERY HAPPY
How did the run feel?
☆ ☆ ☆ ☆ ☆
HARD ⟷ EASY
Water Tracker

DAY 6 Time: Mileage: :
Date: Route: Choice: : Y/N

Distance/Time:
Workout:
Weather:
Takeaways:

Stress/Emotion Tracker
○ ○ ○ ○ ○
VERY SAD ⟷ VERY HAPPY
How did the run feel?
☆ ☆ ☆ ☆ ☆
HARD ⟷ EASY
Water Tracker

DAY 7 Time: Mileage: :
Date: Route: Choice: : Y/N

Distance/Time:
Workout:
Weather:
Takeaways:

Stress/Emotion Tracker
○ ○ ○ ○ ○
VERY SAD ⟷ VERY HAPPY
How did the run feel?
☆ ☆ ☆ ☆ ☆
HARD ⟷ EASY
Water Tracker

"DO WHAT YOU
CAN, WITH
WHAT YOU
HAVE, WHERE
YOU ARE."

— THEODORE ROOSEVELT

SELF-CARE Checklist

	M	T	W	TH	F	SA	SU
Drink a glass of water to start the day	☐	☐	☐	☐	☐	☐	☐
Enjoy your run	☐	☐	☐	☐	☐	☐	☐
Get some fresh air	☐	☐	☐	☐	☐	☐	☐
Have a healthy breakfast	☐	☐	☐	☐	☐	☐	☐
Stretch your body	☐	☐	☐	☐	☐	☐	☐
Enjoy your daily mobility	☐	☐	☐	☐	☐	☐	☐
Enjoy some sunshine	☐	☐	☐	☐	☐	☐	☐
Take hot/cold bath or shower	☐	☐	☐	☐	☐	☐	☐
Read something you enjoy	☐	☐	☐	☐	☐	☐	☐
Play some invigorating music	☐	☐	☐	☐	☐	☐	☐
Disconnect	☐	☐	☐	☐	☐	☐	☐
Eat a healthy snack	☐	☐	☐	☐	☐	☐	☐
Wind down by avoiding bright light at night	☐	☐	☐	☐	☐	☐	☐
Get in bed before 10pm	☐	☐	☐	☐	☐	☐	☐

PHASE 3

TIP: Pushing your pace slightly on the last 15 minutes of your long run can help you practice running through fatigue. Try it! It will help during race-day.

WEEK 13: SPECIFIC

DAY 1 Time: Mileage: :
Date: Route: Choice: : Y/N

Distance/Time:
Workout:
Weather:
Takeaways:

Stress/Emotion Tracker
○ ○ ○ ○ ○
VERY SAD ⟷ VERY HAPPY
How did the run feel?
☆ ☆ ☆ ☆ ☆
HARD ⟷ EASY
Water Tracker

DAY 2 Time: Mileage: :
Date: Route: Choice: : Y/N

Distance/Time:
Workout:
Weather:
Takeaways:

Stress/Emotion Tracker
○ ○ ○ ○ ○
VERY SAD ⟷ VERY HAPPY
How did the run feel?
☆ ☆ ☆ ☆ ☆
HARD ⟷ EASY
Water Tracker

DAY 3 Time: Mileage: :
Date: Route: Choice: : Y/N

Distance/Time:
Workout:
Weather:
Takeaways:

Stress/Emotion Tracker
○ ○ ○ ○ ○
VERY SAD ⟷ VERY HAPPY
How did the run feel?
☆ ☆ ☆ ☆ ☆
HARD ⟷ EASY
Water Tracker

DAY 4 Date: | Time: Route: | Mileage: Choice: | : : Y/N

Distance/Time:

Workout:

Weather:

Takeaways:

Stress/Emotion Tracker
○ ○ ○ ○ ○
VERY SAD ⟷ VERY HAPPY
How did the run feel?
☆ ☆ ☆ ☆ ☆
HARD ⟷ EASY
Water Tracker

DAY 5 Date: | Time: Route: | Mileage: Choice: | : : Y/N

Distance/Time:

Workout:

Weather:

Takeaways:

Stress/Emotion Tracker
○ ○ ○ ○ ○
VERY SAD ⟷ VERY HAPPY
How did the run feel?
☆ ☆ ☆ ☆ ☆
HARD ⟷ EASY
Water Tracker

DAY 6 Date: | Time: Route: | Mileage: Choice: | : : Y/N

Distance/Time:

Workout:

Weather:

Takeaways:

Stress/Emotion Tracker
○ ○ ○ ○ ○
VERY SAD ⟷ VERY HAPPY
How did the run feel?
☆ ☆ ☆ ☆ ☆
HARD ⟷ EASY
Water Tracker

DAY 7 Date: | Time: Route: | Mileage: Choice: | : : Y/N

Distance/Time:

Workout:

Weather:

Takeaways:

Stress/Emotion Tracker
○ ○ ○ ○ ○
VERY SAD ⟷ VERY HAPPY
How did the run feel?
☆ ☆ ☆ ☆ ☆
HARD ⟷ EASY
Water Tracker

"

"THERE IS NO GLORY IN PRACTICE, BUT WITHOUT PRACTICE, THERE IS NO GLORY."

— UNKNOWN

SELF-CARE Checklist

	M	T	W	TH	F	SA	SU
Drink a glass of water to start the day	☐	☐	☐	☐	☐	☐	☐
Enjoy your run	☐	☐	☐	☐	☐	☐	☐
Get some fresh air	☐	☐	☐	☐	☐	☐	☐
Have a healthy breakfast	☐	☐	☐	☐	☐	☐	☐
Stretch your body	☐	☐	☐	☐	☐	☐	☐
Enjoy your daily mobility	☐	☐	☐	☐	☐	☐	☐
Enjoy some sunshine	☐	☐	☐	☐	☐	☐	☐
Take hot/cold bath or shower	☐	☐	☐	☐	☐	☐	☐
Read something you enjoy	☐	☐	☐	☐	☐	☐	☐
Play some invigorating music	☐	☐	☐	☐	☐	☐	☐
Disconnect	☐	☐	☐	☐	☐	☐	☐
Eat a healthy snack	☐	☐	☐	☐	☐	☐	☐
Wind down by avoiding bright light at night	☐	☐	☐	☐	☐	☐	☐
Get in bed before 10pm	☐	☐	☐	☐	☐	☐	☐

Training Notes

Mental Health

Phase 3 Tracker

How was my sleep during the phase?

Approx. hours __________

Get up time __________

How was I feeling throughout this phase?

Great Good Okay Not good Awful

Things I am proud of accomplishing

- Base Run
- Speed Session
- Long Run
- Mobility
- Nutirtion
- Rest and Recovery

Other: __________

How am I feeling right now?

Great Good Okay Not good Awful

Am I satisfied with this day?

I am grateful today for

What I like about myself today

What I managed to do today

What I would like to tell myself for tomorrow

Notes

How and what would I like to feel tomorrow

joy appreciation empowered enthusiasm
fun proud strong active love
passion freedom happiness optimism
belief hope inspired courage interest
amusement gratitude delight relaxed
calm confident curious focused
worthy thrilled self-respecting kind

MILES & MACROS

PHASE 4

TAPER

Absorb Your Training

- Rest.
- Recover.
- Trust in your training.

"CHAMPIONS KEEP PLAYING UNTIL THEY GET IT RIGHT."

— BILLIE JEAN KING

Positive Self Talk and Athletic Performance.

Positive Self-Talk: When you shift your inner dialogue from negative to positive to boost your mental health and outlook on life.

Positive Self-Talk vs. Athletic Performance.

Overcoming negative thoughts will decrease anxiety levels, create excitement, and lead you to a successful athletic performance.

Positive self-talk can be our advocate or our biggest enemy. Effective use of self-talk can improve your performance by helping you regulate your feelings, thoughts, and conserve your energy about the race you have coming up. Positive self-talk can improve your confidence, your focus, performance and motivate you. What motivates you can make you become more productive!

How can you take negative self-talk and make it positive when your emotions and nerves are at an all time high before an upcoming race? Here are some examples below how taking a negative thought and turning it into a positive can be motivating.

CHANGE YOUR NEGATIVE SELF-TALK	TO POSITIVE SELF-TALK
This distance is new to me.	This is an opportunity to learn something.
This workout is too complicated. I am never going to finish!	I'll tackle it from a different angle. I know I can do this. I have trained hard!
What if I fail?	What if this works out?
This is not how I normally do it.	Let's take a chance.
I'm not going to get any better at this.	I'll give it another try.
This is difficult.	Let's break this into smaller steps.
Everyone is better than me.	Being with experienced people will push me.

Talking to yourself negatively will almost ALWAYS result in a poor performance. You have set yourself up for failure before you even tried. Learning to spin that negative self-talk gives you a chance to try your hand at something you're fearful of. Regardless of the result of the experience, the point is – you had the experience!!! This will only set you up for future success.

So, next time you are struggling with negative thoughts, try your best to look for a silver-lining. The more you practice positive self-talk, the more it will become a habit.

PHASE 4

TIP: Taking a collagen supplement 30 to 60 minutes before exercise promotes collagen-building amino acids. This can help promote healing.

WEEK 14: TAPER

DAY 1 Date:	Time: Route:	Mileage: Choice:	: : Y/N
Distance/Time:		Stress/Emotion Tracker ○ ○ ○ ○ ○ VERY SAD ⟷ VERY HAPPY	
Workout:		How did the run feel? ☆ ☆ ☆ ☆ ☆ HARD ⟷ EASY	
Weather:		Water Tracker	
Takeaways:			

DAY 2 Date:	Time: Route:	Mileage: Choice:	: : Y/N
Distance/Time:		Stress/Emotion Tracker ○ ○ ○ ○ ○ VERY SAD ⟷ VERY HAPPY	
Workout:		How did the run feel? ☆ ☆ ☆ ☆ ☆ HARD ⟷ EASY	
Weather:		Water Tracker	
Takeaways:			

DAY 3 Date:	Time: Route:	Mileage: Choice:	: : Y/N
Distance/Time:		Stress/Emotion Tracker ○ ○ ○ ○ ○ VERY SAD ⟷ VERY HAPPY	
Workout:		How did the run feel? ☆ ☆ ☆ ☆ ☆ HARD ⟷ EASY	
Weather:		Water Tracker	
Takeaways:			

DAY 4 Time: Mileage: :
Date: Route: Choice: : Y/N

Distance/Time:
Workout:
Weather:
Takeaways:

Stress/Emotion Tracker
○ ○ ○ ○ ○
VERY SAD ⟷ VERY HAPPY
How did the run feel?
☆ ☆ ☆ ☆ ☆
HARD ⟷ EASY
Water Tracker

DAY 5 Time: Mileage: :
Date: Route: Choice: : Y/N

Distance/Time:
Workout:
Weather:
Takeaways:

Stress/Emotion Tracker
○ ○ ○ ○ ○
VERY SAD ⟷ VERY HAPPY
How did the run feel?
☆ ☆ ☆ ☆ ☆
HARD ⟷ EASY
Water Tracker

DAY 6 Time: Mileage: :
Date: Route: Choice: : Y/N

Distance/Time:
Workout:
Weather:
Takeaways:

Stress/Emotion Tracker
○ ○ ○ ○ ○
VERY SAD ⟷ VERY HAPPY
How did the run feel?
☆ ☆ ☆ ☆ ☆
HARD ⟷ EASY
Water Tracker

DAY 7 Time: Mileage: :
Date: Route: Choice: : Y/N

Distance/Time:
Workout:
Weather:
Takeaways:

Stress/Emotion Tracker
○ ○ ○ ○ ○
VERY SAD ⟷ VERY HAPPY
How did the run feel?
☆ ☆ ☆ ☆ ☆
HARD ⟷ EASY
Water Tracker

"TO GIVE
ANYTHING LESS
THAN YOUR BEST
IS TO SACRIFICE
THE GIFT."

— STEVE PREFONTAINE

SELF-CARE Checklist

	M	T	W	TH	F	SA	SU
Drink a glass of water to start the day	☐	☐	☐	☐	☐	☐	☐
Enjoy your run	☐	☐	☐	☐	☐	☐	☐
Get some fresh air	☐	☐	☐	☐	☐	☐	☐
Have a healthy breakfast	☐	☐	☐	☐	☐	☐	☐
Stretch your body	☐	☐	☐	☐	☐	☐	☐
Enjoy your daily mobility	☐	☐	☐	☐	☐	☐	☐
Enjoy some sunshine	☐	☐	☐	☐	☐	☐	☐
Take hot/cold bath or shower	☐	☐	☐	☐	☐	☐	☐
Read something you enjoy	☐	☐	☐	☐	☐	☐	☐
Play some invigorating music	☐	☐	☐	☐	☐	☐	☐
Disconnect	☐	☐	☐	☐	☐	☐	☐
Eat a healthy snack	☐	☐	☐	☐	☐	☐	☐
Wind down by avoiding bright light at night	☐	☐	☐	☐	☐	☐	☐
Get in bed before 10pm	☐	☐	☐	☐	☐	☐	☐

PHASE 4

TIP: As you get closer to race-day, take time to shift your inner dialogue with positive self-talk. Intentionally doing this will reduce anxiety, create excitement, and improve your athletic performance.

WEEK 15: TAPER

DAY 1 Time: Mileage: :
Date: Route: Choice: : Y/N

Distance/Time:
Workout:
Weather:
Takeaways:

Stress/Emotion Tracker
○ ○ ○ ○ ○
VERY SAD ⟷ VERY HAPPY
How did the run feel?
☆ ☆ ☆ ☆ ☆
HARD ⟷ EASY
Water Tracker

DAY 2 Time: Mileage: :
Date: Route: Choice: : Y/N

Distance/Time:
Workout:
Weather:
Takeaways:

Stress/Emotion Tracker
○ ○ ○ ○ ○
VERY SAD ⟷ VERY HAPPY
How did the run feel?
☆ ☆ ☆ ☆ ☆
HARD ⟷ EASY
Water Tracker

DAY 3 Time: Mileage: :
Date: Route: Choice: : Y/N

Distance/Time:
Workout:
Weather:
Takeaways:

Stress/Emotion Tracker
○ ○ ○ ○ ○
VERY SAD ⟷ VERY HAPPY
How did the run feel?
☆ ☆ ☆ ☆ ☆
HARD ⟷ EASY
Water Tracker

DAY 4
Date:
Time:
Route:
Mileage:
Choice:
:
: Y/N

Distance/Time:

Workout:

Weather:

Takeaways:

Stress/Emotion Tracker
○ ○ ○ ○ ○
VERY SAD ⟷ VERY HAPPY

How did the run feel?
☆ ☆ ☆ ☆ ☆
HARD ⟷ EASY

Water Tracker

DAY 5
Date:
Time:
Route:
Mileage:
Choice:
:
: Y/N

Distance/Time:

Workout:

Weather:

Takeaways:

Stress/Emotion Tracker
○ ○ ○ ○ ○
VERY SAD ⟷ VERY HAPPY

How did the run feel?
☆ ☆ ☆ ☆ ☆
HARD ⟷ EASY

Water Tracker

DAY 6
Date:
Time:
Route:
Mileage:
Choice:
:
: Y/N

Distance/Time:

Workout:

Weather:

Takeaways:

Stress/Emotion Tracker
○ ○ ○ ○ ○
VERY SAD ⟷ VERY HAPPY

How did the run feel?
☆ ☆ ☆ ☆ ☆
HARD ⟷ EASY

Water Tracker

DAY 7
Date:
Time:
Route:
Mileage:
Choice:
:
: Y/N

Distance/Time:

Workout:

Weather:

Takeaways:

Stress/Emotion Tracker
○ ○ ○ ○ ○
VERY SAD ⟷ VERY HAPPY

How did the run feel?
☆ ☆ ☆ ☆ ☆
HARD ⟷ EASY

Water Tracker

"START WHERE
YOU ARE.
USE WHAT
YOU HAVE.
DO WHAT
YOU CAN."

— ARTHUR ASHE

SELF-CARE Checklist

	M	T	W	TH	F	SA	SU
Drink a glass of water to start the day	☐	☐	☐	☐	☐	☐	☐
Enjoy your run	☐	☐	☐	☐	☐	☐	☐
Get some fresh air	☐	☐	☐	☐	☐	☐	☐
Have a healthy breakfast	☐	☐	☐	☐	☐	☐	☐
Stretch your body	☐	☐	☐	☐	☐	☐	☐
Enjoy your daily mobility	☐	☐	☐	☐	☐	☐	☐
Enjoy some sunshine	☐	☐	☐	☐	☐	☐	☐
Take hot/cold bath or shower	☐	☐	☐	☐	☐	☐	☐
Read something you enjoy	☐	☐	☐	☐	☐	☐	☐
Play some invigorating music	☐	☐	☐	☐	☐	☐	☐
Disconnect	☐	☐	☐	☐	☐	☐	☐
Eat a healthy snack	☐	☐	☐	☐	☐	☐	☐
Wind down by avoiding bright light at night	☐	☐	☐	☐	☐	☐	☐
Get in bed before 10pm	☐	☐	☐	☐	☐	☐	☐

PHASE 4

TIP: Train for the terrain your race is on! Specific race-day training is important. Mimic the course terrain, elevation, etc. in your training.

WEEK 16: TAPER

DAY 1 Date:	Time: Route:	Mileage: Choice:	: Y/N
Distance/Time:		**Stress/Emotion Tracker** ○ ○ ○ ○ ○ VERY SAD ⟷ VERY HAPPY	
Workout:		**How did the run feel?** ☆ ☆ ☆ ☆ ☆ HARD ⟷ EASY	
Weather:		**Water Tracker**	
Takeaways:			

DAY 2 Date:	Time: Route:	Mileage: Choice:	: Y/N
Distance/Time:		**Stress/Emotion Tracker** ○ ○ ○ ○ ○ VERY SAD ⟷ VERY HAPPY	
Workout:		**How did the run feel?** ☆ ☆ ☆ ☆ ☆ HARD ⟷ EASY	
Weather:		**Water Tracker**	
Takeaways:			

DAY 3 Date:	Time: Route:	Mileage: Choice:	: Y/N
Distance/Time:		**Stress/Emotion Tracker** ○ ○ ○ ○ ○ VERY SAD ⟷ VERY HAPPY	
Workout:		**How did the run feel?** ☆ ☆ ☆ ☆ ☆ HARD ⟷ EASY	
Weather:		**Water Tracker**	
Takeaways:			

DAY 4
Date:
Time:
Route:
Mileage:
Choice:
:
: Y/N

Distance/Time:
Workout:
Weather:
Takeaways:

Stress/Emotion Tracker
○ ○ ○ ○ ○
VERY SAD ⟷ VERY HAPPY
How did the run feel?
☆ ☆ ☆ ☆ ☆
HARD ⟷ EASY
Water Tracker

DAY 5
Date:
Time:
Route:
Mileage:
Choice:
:
: Y/N

Distance/Time:
Workout:
Weather:
Takeaways:

Stress/Emotion Tracker
○ ○ ○ ○ ○
VERY SAD ⟷ VERY HAPPY
How did the run feel?
☆ ☆ ☆ ☆ ☆
HARD ⟷ EASY
Water Tracker

DAY 6
Date:
Time:
Route:
Mileage:
Choice:
:
: Y/N

Distance/Time:
Workout:
Weather:
Takeaways:

Stress/Emotion Tracker
○ ○ ○ ○ ○
VERY SAD ⟷ VERY HAPPY
How did the run feel?
☆ ☆ ☆ ☆ ☆
HARD ⟷ EASY
Water Tracker

DAY 7
Date:
Time:
Route:
Mileage:
Choice:
:
: Y/N

Distance/Time:
Workout:
Weather:
Takeaways:

Stress/Emotion Tracker
○ ○ ○ ○ ○
VERY SAD ⟷ VERY HAPPY
How did the run feel?
☆ ☆ ☆ ☆ ☆
HARD ⟷ EASY
Water Tracker

Race Day Takeaways

Date:	Time:	Mileage:	:
	Route:	Choice:	: Y/N

Distance/Time:	Stress/Emotion Tracker ○ ○ ○ ○ ○ VERY SAD ⟷ VERY HAPPY
Race Name:	How did the run feel? ☆ ☆ ☆ ☆ ☆ HARD ⟷ EASY
Race Day Weather:	
Did you PR?	Water Tracker

Race Day Takeaways

RACE START TIME

WHAT DID YOU WEAR?

STARTING TEMPERATURE

WHAT DID YOU FUEL WITH?

WHEN DID YOU TAKE FUEL?

DID YOU USE AID STATIONS?

TEMPERATURE MID-RACE

WHAT WERE ISSUES YOU ENCOUNTERED?

HOW WAS YOUR HYDRATION?

WAS THE RACE WELL ORGANIZED?

HOW WAS THE RACE ATOMSPHERE?

FINISH TIME

SELF-CARE Checklist

	M	T	W	TH	F	SA	SU
Drink a glass of water to start the day	☐	☐	☐	☐	☐	☐	☐
Enjoy your run	☐	☐	☐	☐	☐	☐	☐
Get some fresh air	☐	☐	☐	☐	☐	☐	☐
Have a healthy breakfast	☐	☐	☐	☐	☐	☐	☐
Stretch your body	☐	☐	☐	☐	☐	☐	☐
Enjoy your daily mobility	☐	☐	☐	☐	☐	☐	☐
Enjoy some sunshine	☐	☐	☐	☐	☐	☐	☐
Take hot/cold bath or shower	☐	☐	☐	☐	☐	☐	☐
Read something you enjoy	☐	☐	☐	☐	☐	☐	☐
Play some invigorating music	☐	☐	☐	☐	☐	☐	☐
Disconnect	☐	☐	☐	☐	☐	☐	☐
Eat a healthy snack	☐	☐	☐	☐	☐	☐	☐
Wind down by avoiding bright light at night	☐	☐	☐	☐	☐	☐	☐
Get in bed before 10pm	☐	☐	☐	☐	☐	☐	☐

Mental Health

Phase 4 Tracker

How was my sleep during the phase?

Approx. hours ____________

Get up time ____________

How was I feeling throughout this phase?

Great   Good   Okay   Not good   Awful

Things I am proud of accomplishing

- Base Run
- Speed Session
- Long Run
- Mobility
- Nutirtion
- Rest and Recovery

Other: ____

How am I feeling right now?

Great   Good   Okay   Not good   Awful

Am I satisfied with this day?

I am grateful today for

What I like about myself today

What I managed to do today

What I would like to tell myself for tomorrow

Notes

How and what would I like to feel tomorrow

joy appreciation empowered enthusiasm
fun proud strong active love
passion freedom happiness optimism
belief hope inspired courage interest
amusement gratitude delight relaxed
calm confident curious focused
worthy thrilled self-respecting kind

"THE HARDER THE BATTLE, THE SWEETER THE VICTORY."

— LES BROWN

Fuel Before You Are Hungry.

When race season is over, many of you may be taking time to reflect on your race and what you could do better next time. Did you bonk? Did you start to experience cramping? Did the run feel effortless or did it feel exhausting from start to finish?

Whether your next goal is a spring marathon or maybe you are waiting until the next fall season; racing a half, full, or ultra-marathon you will have many progressive long runs integrated into the training plan weekly to help you improve in your endurance for your goal race. In order to achieve these distances, you must fuel correctly.

When it comes to fueling for a race, you don't have to be new to running to have questions. It takes many of us quite a few tries to understand what works best during a long run or race and, at times, learning how to fuel your long runs can feel overwhelming.

How Long Before I Start Fueling?

In general, runners need to add in 30 grams to 60 grams of carbohydrates each hour that they are running when they are running longer than 90 minutes. The timing of your fueling will need to start earlier than 90 minutes into a run. If you wait until 90 minutes to being fueling, by that time your tank will be empty.

Once your tank hits empty it is very hard to recover - if you can recover at all. You should plan to eat 30 grams - 60 grams (depending on your specific body weight/needs) every 45 minutes when you are running longer than 90 minutes. Any long runs greater than 2.5 hours, male or female, consumption of 90 grams of carbohydrates per hour is recommended.

If you are starting from scratch with fueling for your long runs, starting with much smaller quantities of carbohydrates every 45 minutes during your runs may be beneficial to avoid gastrointestinal distress. Start small and work your way up.

But WHY is the timing so important? Our bodies have been continuously working for an extended amount of time and when working for that amount of time we start to run low in glycogen (stored carbohydrates) and get closer to "bonking" or feel the need to stop running at the same intensity. If we fuel ourselves before we start to feel tired and while we are still feeling strong, we can keep our glycogen levels and, in turn, our intensity levels consistent.

It's also important to note that the longer you are moving at a certain effort level, cardiovascular drift occurs. This means that for a constant effort level, the longer you go, there is a gradual increase in heart rate. So by fueling earlier in your run, you are able to absorb carbohydrates better because the need to pump blood (and oxygen) to working muscles is less and the blood flow needed to promote proper carbohydrate digestion is higher.

Remember to start practicing your fueling early into your training. The earlier the better, this way you can try various products and train your gut to take on fuel. Just like you train your legs and your lungs to be strong enough to carry you through a workout, you must train your body to take in calories. If you neglect gut training until race-day, you may experience gastrointestinal distress, cramps, or bonking.

What Should I Fuel With?

When you run long distances, your body relies initially on glycogen as its primary fuel. Glycogen is derived from eating carbohydrates and stored in the muscles and liver for easily accessible, efficient energy.

Running fuel should consist of easily digestible carbohydrates that contain minimal protein, fat, and fiber. While fat is an essential energy source for your body, it takes a while for your body to convert fat into fuel. Protein should be a huge part of your daily diet and post-exercise recovery; however, it is not a primary energy source and, therefore, not a typically essential component of mid-run fueling.

Fueling also consists of hydration. It is important that you take into consideration your hydration strategy for long runs. Chews, gels, sports nutrition beverages, and whole foods may be used to fuel your long runs as these contain those quick digesting carbohydrates. Some athletes use bananas, gummy bears, or home-made energy bites as their fuel.

You should also aim for 300 to 500mg of sodium per hour with 16 to 24 ounces of fluid.

How to Practice Fueling.

Here are some tips on how to start practicing your fueling. Remember it will look different for each runner.

- Fueling needs to be introduced early into your training block. Get used to taking in calories before your long runs are very long.
- Starting early enough allows you to try a variety of flavors and consistencies (gel vs. chew vs. waffle). If you don't like the taste, try out something different.
- If you don't tolerate a product the first time doesn't mean it won't get better. Remember you are actually training your gut as well!
- Practice with what you plan to use on race-day. NEVER try anything new on race-day!
- Practice how you will be carrying your fuel with what you plan to do on race-day.
- Always bring extra fuel just in case you need it.

SAMPLES

Sample Week

Monday	Tuesday	Wednesday	Thursday	Friday	Saturday	Sunday
Base Run	Base Run	Speed Session	Base Run	Rest Day	Long Run	Base Run

Sample Speed

Workout	Intermediate/Half Marathoners	Advanced/Marathoners
Hill Repeats (once every 5 weeks)	25 minutes (Hard burst uphill/ Very easy downhill)	35 minutes (Hard burst uphill/ Very easy downhill)
Threshold Intervals	4 x 4 minutes hard w/ 2 minutes jog between	6 x 4 minutes hard w/ 2 minutes jog between
Dynamic Speed Intervals	6 sets of 1 x 30 sec. > 90 sec. > 30 sec. hard w/ 60 sec. jog between each interval	8 sets of 1 x 30 sec. > 90 sec. > 30 sec. hard w/ 60 sec. jog between each interval
Medium Tempo	1 x 30 minutes hard	1 x 40 minutes hard
Ladder	1 min hard/2 min easy > 2 min hard/3 min easy > 3 min hard/4 min easy > 4 min hard/4 min easy > 4 min hard/3 min easy > 3 min hard/2 min easy > 2 min hard/1 min easy > 1 min hard	1 min hard/2 min easy > 2 min hard/3 min easy > 3 min hard/4 min easy > 4 min hard/5 min easy > 5 min hard/5 min easy > 5 min hard/4 min easy > 4 min hard/4 min easy > 3 min hard/3 min easy > 2 min hard/2 min easy > 1 min hard

About Your Trainer

Lauren Burdick is a certified sports nutrition consultant and certified running coach.

Lauren is co-owner of Miles & Macros. LLC, a small business established in 2021, with her husband, Jared. They both live in Fayetteville, NY with their two doodles (the kids).

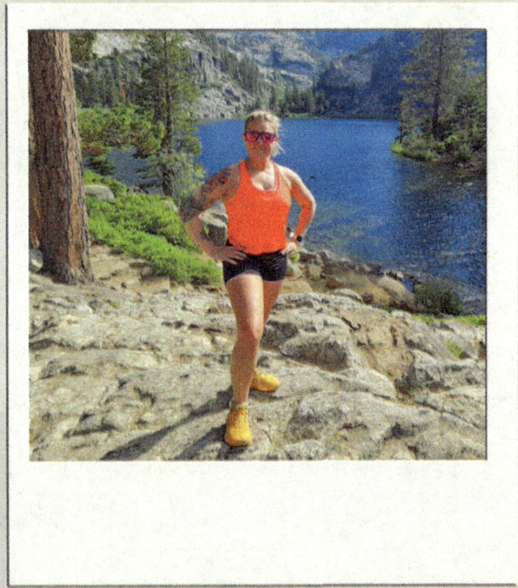

RUN

About Our Business

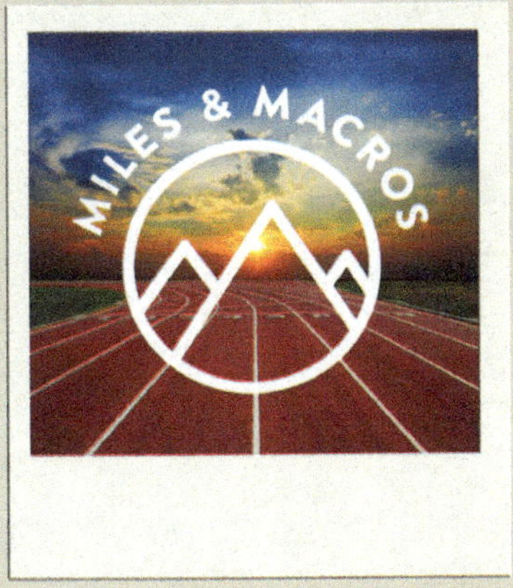

Miles & Macros, LLC specializes in tailored fitness services to help meet your individual goals. Our programs feature half marathon and marathon running, cycling, and strength workouts, all available on our convenient mobile app for both in-person, group, and virtual options.

We believe that in order to run or cycle at your best, you will need a great team around to support you and be in your corner. We believe that one of the most important things a coach can bring to the athlete is perspective and clarity. Life can be stressful and demanding on its own and additional pressures to perform can often times be offloaded to the coach.

Discover a new level of fitness today with Miles & Macros by scanning this QR code or going to www.milesandmacros.net!

Made in United States
North Haven, CT
10 November 2026

22091335R00068